BEAUTY
LIVES

BUILDING UP ANATOMY

JERRICA RASHAD WHITTIER

WRITERS REPUBLIC L.L.C.
515 Summit Ave. Unit R1
Union City, NJ 07087, USA

Website: *www.writersrepublic.com*
Hotline: *1-877-656-6838*
Email: *info@writersrepublic.com*

Ordering Information:
Quantity sales. Special discounts are available on quantity purchases by corporations, associations, and others. For details, contact the publisher at the address above.

Library of Congress Control Number: 2020941726
ISBN-13:   978-1-64620-464-9   [Paperback Edition]
                  978-1-64620-465-6   [Digital Edition]

Rev. date: 06/29/0000

CONTENTS

I am thankful that our Heavenly Father gave me a gift to share, and all the years of research and culture to heal others and self.

We, as a people, usually have many questions based on a natural curiosity on how to restore our body's health. We notice in our own perceptions that the products and services promoted and being advertised are not usually what's best for us. A lot of us have and had questions growing up in class that were unanswered due to the lack of research of even the teacher. Well I took the time to save you some time and researched different sectors on how to rebuild your anatomy's immune system. This book will heal you from the inside out and outside in. I know you've heard the term "you are what you eat". Well fortunately and unfortunately it was true. I know that when we reach a certain age in life we often feel like "oh I'm grown now I can do whatever I want to do". Well yes you do have free will to do whatever you want to do but nevertheless that doesn't mean you don't have a consequence. There are good consequences and there are bad consequences even in nature. If you had a car and you did not put the proper fuel, oil and water in your car it would not operate in the way that it should operate, it would fail you. Well your body is a lot like a car. If you do not put in the Necessities to keep that body running functionally it will fail you. Life brings life. Positive makes a positive. Death brings death. Negative equals another negative. These examples are simple formulas that were most likely discovered to you during your kindergarten through 8th grade sessions of schooling. But one thing we've known no matter what is that facts or facts. If you had a chance to find out things that could heal your asthma, heal your skin, grow your hair and build your immune system to the point where it can withstand anything that's attacking it. What I'm saying to you is its time to build an immune system shield. These are all options and choices to choose from that will build your immune system and make it Invincible to viruses and diseases that you can and cannot see. We Are chameleons and Survivors by Nature but we have been practicing acts that is against nature based on a long line of things and events that have happened throughout the time lines. This is not the time to become distracted nor panic, it's time to heal our families and execute. It's time to get back to the basics. What greater way then the Start of building and healing our immune system.

FRUIT FOR THOUGHT

Apples are not just pretty in colors or tasty treats. They have all types of healing and growth vitals for the anatomy. Apples are a fruit for thoughts and assist with the elevation growth and maturity in the body. It has been my experience after eating an apple, my mind would create new vibrant idea solutions of how to simplify and conquer problems that where at first seemed to be too hard or not feasible at the time. After eating apples I was now invincible in the mind, all of a sudden everything was a formulated solution and I was the solution.

Facts of an apple according to healthline.com, apples have healing properties such as manganese, copper, and the vitamins A, E, B1, B2, and B6. Apples may aid weight loss in several ways. They're also particularly filling due to their high fiber content. Apples are also a rich source of polyphenols. Apples promote heart health in several ways. Eating apples is linked to a lower risk of type 2 diabetes. This is possibly due to their polyphenol antioxidant content. The type of fiber in apples feeds good bacteria and may be the reason they protect against obesity, heart disease, and type 2 diabetes. Apples have several naturally occurring compounds that may help fight cancer. Observational studies have linked them to a lower risk of cancer and death from cancer. Antioxidant-rich apples may help protect your lungs from oxidative damage. Apples contain antioxidant and anti-inflammatory compounds that may help regulate immune responses and protect against asthma. The antioxidant and anti-inflammatory compounds in apples may promote bone health. What's more, eating fruit may help preserve bone mass as you age. Apples contain compounds that may help protect your stomach lining from injury due to NSAID painkillers. According to animal studies, apple juice may help prevent the decline of neurotransmitters that are involved in memory. They're high in soluble fiber, which helps lower cholesterol. They also have polyphenols, which are linked to lower blood pressure and stroke risk. For those that need a little more assist polyphenols according to Health line through the google search engine, Polyphenols are micronutrients that we get through certain plant-based foods. They're packed with antioxidants and potential health benefits. It's thought that polyphenols can improve or help treat digestion issues, weight management difficulties, diabetes, neurodegenerative disease, and cardiovascular disease. Let's just say eating an apple a day and the growing of an apple tree is a valuable problem fixer. Apples heal the reproduction system, stops hunger, grants wisdom, allows for fresh energy. Apples protect your body from the invading seen and unseen bacteria.

Get creative when bringing fruits and Veggies to your children, here's a few tips or ideas to start you off. Healthyhappylife.com really put in time and efforts on how to use them apples they have managed to create; caramel apple pie, applesauce, caramel apples, they even put them in different salads with special seasonings, stuffed apple turnover in a skillet sounds yummy right. There are many uses for apples and you can make them in different ways: you can make them in desserts, you can make them in meals, and you can even make them in small snacks. There is never an excuse to not appreciate the apple, fruit for thought.

Pears. I found accordingly to Medical news today articles they state that pears are rich in essential antioxidants, plant compounds, and dietary fiber. They pack all of these nutrients in a fat free, cholesterol free, 100 calorie package. As part of a balanced, nutritious diet, consuming pears could support weight loss and reduce a person's risk of cancer, diabetes, and heart disease. Also using Google engine you can find health.com also speaks out about pears saying this anti-aging fruit gives your skin a big beauty boost, whether you eat it or apply it! Pears are full of fiber, a crucial nutrient for your skin. ... "Pears also have vitamin C, which fights free radicals." So crunching on a Bosc or Bartlett a day may help keep the wrinkles away. You hear that Queens and Kings no more worrying about aging get you some pears. According to organicfacts.net, the skin, eye, and hair care can be added by the pear. Also if you look more in their table of contents you will find a chapter on each of these following topics in depth on how Health Benefits of Pears Optimize Digestion, Weight Loss, and Antioxidant Activity. Pears offer Anticancer Potential, Boost Immunity, Improve Heart Health and Speeds Healing. Wow! Improves Circulation, Reduce Inflammation, Improves Health, and Skin & Hair Care. Get you some seeds of a pear and grow you a pear tree it's like an acting agent for regenerating.

Check out recipes for pears;

https://www.veganricha.com/vegan-pear
https://simple-veganista.com/rustic-apple-pear-crisp/

Now get creative.

Avocado fruit is botanically a large berry containing a single large seed according to Wikipedia. According to healthline.com avocados are high in; Vitamin K: 26% of the daily value also Folate: 20%, Vitamin C: 17%, Potassium: 14%, Vitamin B5: 14%, Vitamin B6: 13%, Vitamin E: 10%. It also contains small amounts of magnesium, manganese, copper, iron, zinc, phosphorous and vitamins A, B1 (thiamine),

B2 (riboflavin) and B3 (niacin).Potassium is an important mineral that most people don't get enough of. Avocados are very high in potassium, which should support healthy blood pressure Avocados and avocado oil are high in monounsaturated oleic acid, a heart-healthy fatty acid that is believed to be one of the main reasons for the health benefits of olive oil. Avocados tend to be rich in fiber — about 7% by weight, which is very high compared to most other foods. Fiber may have important benefits for weight loss and metabolic health. Numerous studies have shown that eating avocado can improve heart disease risk factors like total, "bad" LDL and "good" HDL cholesterol, as well as blood triglycerides. One dietary survey found that people who ate avocados had a much higher nutrient intake and a lower risk of metabolic syndrome. Studies have shown that eating avocado or avocado oil with vegetables can dramatically increase the number of antioxidants you take in. Avocados are high in antioxidants, including lutein and zeaxanthin. These nutrients are very important for eye health and lower your risk of macular degeneration and cataracts. Some test-tube studies have shown that nutrients in avocados may have benefits in preventing prostate cancer and lowering side effects of chemotherapy. However, human-based research is lacking. Studies have shown that avocado and soybean oil extracts can significantly reduce symptoms of osteoarthritis. Avocados may aid weight loss by keeping you full longer and making you eat fewer calories. They're also high in fiber and low in carbs, which may promote weight loss. Avocados have a creamy, rich, fatty texture and blend well with other ingredients. Therefore, it's easy to add this fruit to your diet. Using lemon juice may prevent cut avocados from browning quickly. We got to give it up to healthline. com they definitely took the time to let us know how beautiful and appreciative we should be of the avocado. Avocado is a Healer for the body inside and out every stores all that has been lost inside the body and outside the body. Here are so fun recipes to incorporate with the avocado. I really love avocado with crackers with salads, on tacos, quesadillas. Avocado is really a variety of things you can do with. It is a delicious fruit which is crazy because I thought it was a vegetable. You can find great recipes on these following sites;

www.Live kindly. Com or www.peta.org

Blueberries, According to Medical news today, the fiber, potassium, folate, vitamin C, vitamin B6, and phytonutrient content in blueberries supports heart health. The absence of cholesterol from blueberries is also beneficial to the heart. Fiber content helps to reduce the total amount of cholesterol in the blood and decrease the risk of heart disease. Accordingly to www.sciencedaily.com, eating blueberries every day improves heart health. Summary: Eating a cup of blueberries a day reduces risk factors for cardiovascular disease -- according to a new study. Eating 150g of blueberries daily reduces the risk of cardiovascular disease by up to 15 per cent. Webmd.com says that blueberries are a superfood. Webmd.com also says Packed with antioxidants and phytoflavinoids, these berries are also high in potassium and vitamin C, making them the top choice of doctors and nutritionists. Not only can they lower your risk of heart disease and cancer, they are also anti-inflammatory. Healthline.com says that blueberries are the king of all antioxidant fruits. They also state that Blueberries have the highest antioxidant capacity of all the popular fruits and vegetables. Flavonoids appear to be the berries' antioxidant with the greatest impact. Healthline. com offers information facts on several studies suggest that blueberries and blueberry juice reduce DNA damage, which is a leading driver of aging and cancer. The antioxidants in blueberries seem to benefit your brain by aiding brain function and delaying mental decline. Several studies demonstrate that blueberries have anti-diabetes effects, improving insulin sensitivity and lowering blood sugar levels. Like cranberries, blueberries contain substances that can prevent certain bacteria from binding to the wall of your bladder, which may help prevent UTIs. One study suggests that blueberries may aid muscle recovery after strenuous exercise, though more research is needed. Blueberries are incredibly healthy and nutritious. You can make blueberry pie, blueberry muffins, blueberry salad there's so many ways to eat blueberries. Here are some websites 4 blueberry recipes;

https://mayihavethatrecipe.com/vegan-blueberry-crumble/

https://www.mydarlingvegan.com/vegan-blueberry-muffins/

https://www.exceedinglyvegan.com/vegan-recipes/baking-desserts/easy-vegan-blueberry-cake

Walnuts accordingly to brain IQ Walnuts are the top nut for brain health. They have a significantly high concentration of DHA, a type of Omega-3 fatty acid. Among other things, DHA has been shown to protect brain health in newborns, improve cognitive performance in adults, and prevent or ameliorate age-related cognitive decline. Here are some walnut recipes fat delicious try them out or create your own.

https://www.vnutritionandwellness.com/walnut-meat-tacos/

https://minimalistbaker.com/10-minute-raw-vegan-taco-meat/

Papaya Lowers cholesterol. Papaya is rich in fibre, Vitamin C and antioxidants which helps in weight loss and boosts your immunity. It's been said to be amazing for diabetics and protects against pain.

Check out this amazing salad Papaya dish at https://minimalistbaker.com/vegan-papaya-salad

Honeydew accordingly to research shows provides you with natural sugars that will continue to fuel your cells throughout the day. It also is low in fat and contains several key vitamins and minerals, such as: Vitamin C: proven to boost your immune system, as well as give you healthy skin, strengthen tissues, and promote healthy brain function.

Pineapple are filled with bromelain, an enzyme that helps the body digest proteins.

Plums have an excellent source of vitamins, minerals, fiber and antioxidants. They also reduce the risk of many chronic diseases, such as osteoporosis, cancer, heart disease and diabetes.

Tomatoes reduce the risk of heart disease and cancer. They contain high amounts of vitamin C, potassium, folate, and vitamin K.

Nectarines has a lot of fiber, vitamin A, vitamin C, and potassium.

Jackfruit contains vitamin C, potassium, dietary fiber, and traces of other vitamins and minerals. In the skin, seeds, and other parts of the plant may have the potential to treat or prevent a number of health conditions. Jackfruit has been used as a tasty cultured meat substitute.

Mango fighting cancer, cholesterol level, cleansing skin, diabetes alkalizing your body. Also assists with losing weight. Mango is an Aphrodisiac fruit that also is for healing eyes.

Strawberries have vitamin C and manganese and also contain good daily intake amounts of folate (vitamin B9) and potassium.

Peaches are helps for digestion and boost your immune system. They firm up your skin too. Peaches protect your eyesight. It's said to lower cancer risk. Peaches might promote brain health and blood pressure control and de-bloating.

Coconut has an amazing boost in good Cholesterol. It's great for Blood Sugar and Diabetes health. Studied reveal Coconut is great for healing Alzheimer's disease. Researchers have also determined it helps stop Heart Disease and High Blood Pressure. This amazing fruit helps heals the Liver and boosts Energy. Coconut Assists with Digestion. Studies show it heals wounds and Burns.

Cranberries is known to be a superfood due to their high nutrient and antioxidant content. It's a great find that the nutrients in cranberries is known to lower the probability of a urinary tract infection (UTI), the prevention of certain types of cancer, and improvement of the immune system functions.

Cacao has been found to have anti-inflammatory properties and may reduce risk of diabetes. Raw cacao contains magnesium, calcium, iron, zinc, copper, potassium, and manganese A Cacao also known as cocoa pod (fruit) to Americans, has a rough leathery rind about 3 cm thick (this varies with the origin and variety of pod). The plant is thought of as a fruit plant. The bean itself is a seed and a seed technically is a nut. So it comes from the nut inside the fruit. It's made to make chocolate.

Check out https://youtu.be/I05PXP5hysQ. It's amazing what's not being taught all over the world.

When you are able to think clearly because you have a healthy, happy and creative brain you have obtained the proper Energies you need to where you can do all things great positive creative and to overcome adversities.

-Jerrica Whittier

CHAPTER

2

FOODS TO BUILD THE IMMUNE SYSTEM

We tend to live busy lives and are usually not able to really just relax and focus on how we can heal our families due to the constant distractions we most of the time we sit at home and we Google about miscellaneous things took the time to Google some very strong immune system boosters and healers such as:

Lemons are high in vitamin C, a natural antioxidant which enhances the immune system and has antiviral and antibacterial properties. However, apart from supporting the immune system and tasting good, lemons have many other purported benefits and uses: Prevents bacterial growth and infections, Relieves nausea

Honey antioxidant and antibacterial properties help improve the digestive system and boost immunity. It is also a powerhouse of antioxidants, which are very effective for the removal of free radicals from the body.

Onions are packed with immune-boosting nutrients like selenium, sulfur compounds, zinc, and vitamin C. In addition, they are one of the best sources of quercetin, a potent flavonoid, and antioxidant that has antiviral properties as well as histamine regulating effects

Garlic can boost immune function. It contains compounds that help the immune system fight germs (5, 6). Whole garlic contains a compound called Allicin. When garlic is crushed or chewed, this compound turns into Allicin (with a c), the main active ingredient in garlic.

Basil contains natural antibacterial properties. If you're looking for a natural way to boost your immune system or fight off pre-existing infections, basil may do the trick! Basil extract has even been shown to help in inhibiting resistant strains of bacteria that are unable to respond to antibiotics.

Echinacea, Extracts of echinacea do seem to have an effect on the immune system, your body's defense against germs. Research shows it increases the number of white blood cells, which fight infections. A review of more than a dozen studies, published in 2014, found the herbal remedy had a very slight benefit in preventing colds.

Elderberry. The berries and flowers of elderberry are packed with antioxidants and vitamins that may boost your immune system. They can help tame inflammation, lessen stress, and help protect your heart, too. Some experts recommend elderberry to help prevent and ease cold and flu symptoms.

Andrographis is most widely used to treat cold and flu symptoms. Andrographis is also said to act as a natural immune-booster. The herb is also used to treat certain other conditions.

Astragalus contains beneficial plant compounds that may enhance your immune system. The primary role of your immune system is to protect your body against harmful invaders, including bacteria, germs and viruses that can cause illness

Burdock Root is powerful antioxidants, including quercetin, luteolin, and phenolic acids. Antioxidants protect cells in the body from damage due to free radicals. It's used to purify the blood, reduce inflammation and heal cancer.

Ginger is a strong antioxidant that has been shown to naturally boost the immune system. It contains tons of vitamins, some of which are magnesium, iron, zinc, and calcium. Ginger helps kill cold viruses and has been said to combat chills and fever

Broccoli Phytochemicals in broccoli are good for the immune system. They include glucobrassicin; carotenoids, such as zeaxanthin and beta-carotene; and kaempferol, a flavonoid.

Spinach it's rich in vitamin C. It's also packed with numerous antioxidants and beta carotene, which may increase the infection-fighting ability of our immune systems.

Sweet potatoes are rich in beta carotene — a carotenoid that converts into vitamin A — which helps boost the immune system and lower the risk for various diseases. This antioxidant helps protect the body from free radicals and may lower your risk for heart disease and cancer.

Watermelon is an immune-boosting fruit. One 2-cup serving of watermelon has 270 mg of potassium, 30% of the daily value of vitamin A, and 25% of the value of vitamin C. Calories in watermelon aren't much at all. One 2-cup serving of watermelon has just 80 calories. Watermelon also provides vitamin B6 and glutathione.

Kiwi are nutrient-dense and full of vitamin C. In fact, just 1 cup of kiwi provides about 273 percent of your daily recommended value. Vitamin C is an essential nutrient when it comes to boosting your immune system to ward off disease.

Acai berry fruit is high in anthocyanins. These flavonoid molecules are very potent antioxidants. They combat oxidative stress in the body by mopping up free radicals. Antioxidants are credited with boosting immunity and lowering inflammation in the body

Limes high in vitamin C, a nutrient that may help boost your immune system. Besides vitamin C, limes are also a great source of antioxidants, which help strengthen your immune system by defending cells against free radical damage (

Oranges and grapefruit Vitamin C has antioxidant and other properties that protect your cells from substances that damage the body. A deficiency of vitamin C can lead to delayed wound healing, inability to properly fight infections, and impaired immune response.

The vitamin C and carotenoids in Dragon fruit may boost your immune system and prevent infection by protecting your white blood cells from damage (26, 27). ... Summary Dragon fruit's high supply of vitamin C and carotenoids may offer immune-boosting properties.

Kale. Greens such as kale, spinach, and Swiss chard are immune-boosting foods that contain high levels of vitamin C, which not only packs a powerful antioxidant punch, it helps fight off infection and regenerate other antioxidants in the body, including vitamin E. They also contain folate, another immune booster.

We as individuals and some that are head of households and we are responsible Fort healing our bodies we must not leave healing our bodies to another individual without proper research and proper care.

-Jerrica Whittier

CHAPTER 3

THICKENING OF THE BLOOD

Fruits and foods that are high in potassium vitamin K or blood thickeners here are some blood thickness that will heal those that are suffering from thin blood. They are as follows:

Kiwi are filled with vitals K, vitamin E, folate, and potassium. They are a great source of fiber.

Plantains A, C, and B-6, and the minerals magnesium and potassium.

Beans of different sorts such as kidney, soy and beans black beans

Peanuts protein, and fiber. They also contain plenty of potassium, phosphorous, magnesium, and

B vitamins. Peanuts are nutrient-rich and low in carbohydrates.

Bananas contains potassium, manganese, and also help with the digestive system. It has been said that bananas help grant you energy.

Bok choy is an excellent source of vitamin C, vitamin K, vitamin A, and beta-carotene. It is a very good source of folate, calcium, and vitamin B6 as well.

Blueberries are great for a natural high energy and blood flow. It's also great for constipation. It contains fiber, potassium, folate, vitamin C, vitamin B6, and phytonutrient. This tasteful delicious treat has been said to protect your DNA as a whole. I always suggest to research, research, and research for yourself. It helps your own mind to confirm truths.

Carrots are a good source of beta carotene, fiber, vitamin K1, potassium, and antioxidants. They also have a number of health benefits. They're a weight-loss-friendly food and have been linked to lower cholesterol levels and improved eye health.

Sweet potatoes are a great source of fiber, vitamins, and minerals. Promote stomach Health. The fiber and antioxidants in sweet potatoes are needed for overall health. It has cancer-fighting nutrition. Sweet potatoes also helps with healthy vision and enhances brain function. Sweet potatoes support your Immune system shield.

Grapes the nutrients in grapes may help protect against cancer, eye problems, cardiovascular disease, and other health conditions. Resveratrol is a key nutrient in grapes that may offer health benefits. Grapes are a good source of fiber, potassium, and a range of vitamins and other minerals.

Doing some research I've came across, according to drugs.com, Foods that contain vitamin K are dark green leafy vegetables have the highest amounts of vitamin K. Foods that contain vitamin K Are found in foods with more than 100 mcg per serving:

½ cup of cooked kale (531 mcg)
½ cup of cooked spinach (444 mcg)
½ cup of cooked collard greens (418 mcg)
1 cup of cooked broccoli (220 mcg)

1 cup of cooked brussels sprouts (219 mcg)

1 cup of raw collard greens (184 mcg)

1 cup of raw spinach (145 mcg)

1 cup of raw endive (116 mcg)

Foods with 50 to 100 mcg per serving:

1 cup of raw broccoli (89 mcg)

½ cup of cooked cabbage (82 mcg)

1 cup of green leaf lettuce (71 mcg)

1 cup of romaine lettuce (57 mcg)

Foods with 15 to 50 mcg per serving:

4 spears of asparagus (48 mcg)

1 medium kiwi fruit (31 mcg)

1 cup of raw blackberries or blueberries (29 mcg)

1 cup of red or green grapes (23 mcg)

½ cup of cooked peas (19 mcg)

CHAPTER 4

HEALING THICK BLOOD USING BLOOD THINNERS

Have you ever got a charley horse or had blood stuck in one spot and wanted to know "what do I do to ease this pain?" "How do I regulate this regulate the blood throughout my body?" Well here are a few tips on foods that thin the blood.

Newstoday.com puts us up on reality here are some of their in my found research for thinning blood Healers;

Turmeric's curcumin that has anti-inflammatory and blood-thinning or anticoagulant properties. A study published in 2012 suggests that taking a daily dose of turmeric spice may help people maintain the anticoagulant status of their blood.

Ginger. Anti-inflammatory spice that may stop blood clotting. It contains a natural acid called salicylate. Aspirin (acetylsalicylic acid) is a synthetic derivative of salicylate and a potent blood thinner.

Burdock Root purifies blood, reduces inflammation and has been researched to prevent cancer.

Cayenne peppers. Capsaicin promotes blood flow to tissues by lowering blood pressure and stimulating the release of nitric oxide and other vasodilators.

Vitamin E. reduces blood clotting in a few different ways. These effects depend on the amount of vitamin E that a person takes. The National Institutes of Health's Office of Dietary Supplements suggest that people who are taking blood-thinning drugs should avoid taking large doses of vitamin E.

Garlic. Some research reports that odorless garlic powder demonstrates antithrombotic activities. An antithrombotic agent is a substance that reduces blood clot formation. Another review of several studies on garlic suggests that it may thin the blood, although the effects are small and short-lived.

Cassia cinnamon contains coumarin, a powerful blood-thinning agent. Warfarin, the most commonly used blood-thinning drug, is derived from coumarin. It may be best to stick to small amounts of cinnamon in the diet in addition to using other natural blood thinners.

Ginkgo Biloba Extract (GBE) is known to thin the blood and increase blood flow. This is particularly helpful in the small capillaries of the brain, eyes and ears and is just one of a number of reasons why ginkgo is helpful for tinnitus. ... In this paper I refer to three common blood thinners: Coumadin, Plavix and aspirin.

Grape seed extract can potentially affect medications broken down by the liver. ... Anticoagulants (blood thinners): Grape seed extract may act as a blood thinner, and could increase the risk of bleeding if taken with other blood thinners such as warfarin (Coumadin), clopidogrel (Plavix), or aspirin.

5

LET'S HEAL OUR EYESIGHT WITH FOOD

K iwi contains more vitamin C and contains the pigments zeaxanthin and lutein (lutein is often known as the "eye vitamin").

Sweet Potatoes. These orange tubers are a good source of beta carotene. Your body converts beta carotene to vitamin A, a nutrient that helps prevent dry eyes and night blindness. Beta carotene and vitamin A also may help reduce the risk eye infections. Eat right.com

Kale has the antioxidants lutein and zeaxanthin, also found in eggs and other foods. These nutrients may help to prevent serious eye conditions such as age-related macular degeneration and cataracts.

Nuts Almonds, peanuts, pistachios, and cashews are some of the various nuts that are good for the eyes. Nuts are rich in omega-3 fatty acids and vitamin E, which boost your eye health and protect the eye's cells from "free radicals" that could break down the eye's tissue8. (20/20 on site blog)

Herbs helps soothe itchy eyes and conjunctivitis. . . Gingko Biloba: This herb can reduce the risks of glaucoma and macular degeneration by acting as a cerebro-spinal dilator. Fennel: Fennel is said to be particularly helpful for watery and inflamed eyes.

Grapefruit Just a single eight ounce glass of grapefruit juice or eating one grapefruit per day is enough to help maintain your vision and fight off the ravages of eye strain, aging, and other stressors that can chip away at your vision. If you're looking for more eye sight recipes, I suggest this website www.halegroves. com/blog/3-health-benefits-of-eating-grapefruits/

Orange-colored fruits and vegetables -- like sweet potatoes, carrots, cantaloupe, mangos, and apricots -- are high in beta-carotene, a form of vitamin A that helps with night vision, your eyes' ability to adjust to darkness

You can find a lot of more information (if you're a junkie like me) at https://www.webmd.com/eye-health/ss/slideshow-eyes-sight-foods.

CHAPTER 6

KEEPING THE BODY HYDRATED THE ALKALINE DIET

According to webmd.com and there research the alkaline diet claims to help your body maintain its blood pH level. In fact, nothing you eat is going to substantially change the pH of your blood. Your body works to keep that level constant

Decades of research from different doctors and scientists show that alkaline is a necessary component 2 survival of the human body.

According to a healthline.com, the human body is built to naturally maintain a healthy balance of acidity and alkalinity. The lungs and kidneys play a key role in this process. A normal blood pH level is

7.40 on a scale of 0 to 14, where 0 is the most acidic and 14 is the most basic. This value can vary slightly in either direction

High alkaline foods can be found Cody Martin that's an everyday supermarkets.

Avocados, lemons, broccoli are considered high in alkaline. Apples, bananas pineapples are great intakes for alkaline. Grapes, coconuts and limes are examples of high in alkaline on the PH scale.

Like most of us being curious, I started researching through Google because I had to find out exactly what was the meaning of ph and what it stood for. Its simple definition was simple but not so simple. It basically is the measure of acidity or alkalinity of water soluble substances (pH stands for 'potential of Hydrogen'). A pH value is a number from 1 to 14, with 7 as the middle (neutral) point. Values below 7 indicate acidity which increases as the number decreases, 1 being the most acidic.

Water is high in alkaline. Some areas and countries offer higher pH in there alkaline water. Alkaline water has a higher pH level than regular drinking water. Because of this, some advocates of alkaline water believe it can neutralize the acid in your body. The most common drinking water generally has a neutral pH of 7. Alkaline water usually have a potential of hydrogen number of 8. Examples of high pH water that can be found in stores are Smart Water, Life Water, Core Water and there are many more that can be found per store. Your body gives off alerts that let you know just how much you need of a certain object our food or water. Trust your body when it says it's enough too much. Anything too much is obviously isn't good, where you can balance yourself how to know if your body has enough alkaline with just taking one cup, at the most 8oz of alkaline water. Measure your intake of alkaline water by your personal dehydration.

Sweet potatoes and regular potatoes are high in their pH balance. Sweet potatoes sit on a scale of a 5.6. Regular potatoes such as red russett and other potatoes sit on a scale of 5.4 to 5.9. if you want to boost your immune system I totally suggest sweet potatoes are regular potatoes or even red potatoes just get you some good potatoes. There's nothing wrong with starting your own garden and planting potatoes. Not only will you never go hungry or your family but it will boost your immune system. Also they will protect you from viruses and diseases. Some people start their Garden off growing potatoes and it ends up becoming a trade for income or finances. Alkaline is valuable to every living being it's time to immune up and get on the alkaline diet.

CHAPTER 7

STARCHES WHAT THEY DO FOR THE BODY

During the different time zones throughout the millennium, our ancestors have found different solutions to healing the body using starches. Now I know a lot of us that are busy with work life might have questions like what exactly are starches and what are they good for. Well we usually use starches in our everyday life believe It or not. Starches have been used for several different ways of healing inside and outside the body. You can use rice water, potato water for growing your hair crazy right. We have several different home remedies that you can choose from. Starches have been found in rice, grains, herbs, fruits and veggies. It's been my personal experience that I've noticed that starches are in onions rice and grains. On this new journey to healing our immune system I've took extra time to research to compare and contrast, to be able to document how and why starches heal the body.

People long before us have researched different foods. Foods that carry Starch are Starchy foods include peas, corn, potatoes, beans, pasta, rice and grains. Starches are a more concentrated source of carbohydrates and calories than fruits, non-starchy vegetables but many of them are excellent sources of fiber, vitamins, minerals and phytonutrients. Phytonutrients also called phytochemicals, are chemicals produced by plants. ... Phytonutrients can also provide significant benefits for humans who eat plant foods. Phytonutrient-rich foods include colorful fruits and vegetables, legumes, nuts, tea, whole grains and many spices. You can also continue research on starchy foods on Google search always trust your own research, compare and contrast what fits your family needs.

8 HOME REMEDIES TO HEAL THE IMMUNE SYSTEM

A lot of the foods that we eat everyday are Heelers for the immune system. Ancestors like I grandmother is Grandfather's used to do certain things at home that prevented us from going to the hospital and most of the time we didn't get sick we were healed by home remedies.

Some of home remedies I use I've found to be very useful and 100% accurate. I use them for everyday issues such as toothaches, common cold, and building the immune system.

Toothaches can cause the body to go into shock. Toothaches can be caused by bacteria and the mouth holding viruses. Viruses in the mouth can cause the immune system to break down. Get you a lemon slices, 1 orange peel and a lime slice in a bottle of water will get rid of any bad tooth. Also cayenne pepper and peroxide gets rid of pain immediately from a toothache. Cloves the herb gets rid of tooth aches. Also baking soda Kanye pepper and peroxide makes for a great toothpaste and mouthwash for healthy teeth and mouth.

If you got the common cold don't be upset anymore I got a great remedy onions. I usually do red onions but you can do white onions if you prefer. Boil you two onions in some sea salt water and basil. Let it cool down to warm hot temperature then put it in a cup and drink it like a tea. This remedy will reboot your immune system and fight viruses off of your body. The onion method also heals the immune system and builds it.

Grapefruit, grapefruit, grapefruit! Is a great healer for the immune system!

A good susta of mine Velvet M. Clark alerted me that Ginger and warm water heals the cramps ladies!!!

Most of us know about the green tea and black tea method. There are many teas to choose from like. Chamomile Tea. Peppermint tea is also good for fighting viruses. Ginger tea is an inquiring taste but it's healthy and it fights disease. Hibiscus Tea. ... I love!!!! Echinacea Tea, Rooibos Tea and Sage Tea are great boosters and fights anything attacking your immune system. Local Honey is a huge Healer for the immune system to try as a sweetener for your tea. Also try citrus fruits like lemons, oranges, or lime slices in your tea.

CHAPTER 9

VITAMINS ARE NECESSARY FOR THE IMMUNE SYSTEM

Building your immune system has a lot to do with the vitals and minerals you put into your body. Your body is much like a machine for an example most like a car. A car needs gas to drive, a car needs engine oil for the engine to work. A car needs transmission oil for the transmission to work. Your body needs different minerals and vitals to keep it regenerating and working functionally. To fight unseen bacteria you must build your body to shield your insides from harm. The vitamins necessary for the body immune system are as follows;

WebMD tells us that Vitamin C known as ascorbic acid, is necessary for the growth, development and repair of all body tissues. It's involved in many body functions, including formation of collagen, absorption of iron, the immune system, wound healing, and the maintenance of cartilage, bones, and teeth. Vitamin c foods are kiwis, cantaloupe, broccoli, kale, oranges, papaya, red, green or yellow pepper, sweet potatoes and strawberries.

More research gives info on Vitamin E. Vitamin E is a fat-soluble nutrient found in many foods. In the body, it acts as an antioxidant, helping to protect cells from the damage caused by free radicals. Free radicals are compounds formed when our bodies convert the food we eat into energy. Vitamin E foods are avocado, spinach, almonds, leafy vegetables, asparagus, nuts, beans and beets.

Vitamin A is important for normal vision, the immune system, and reproduction. Vitamin A helps the heart, lungs, kidneys, and other organs work properly. Vitamin A foods are carrot, spinach, cantaloupe, sweet potatoes, broccoli, squash, apricot, mango, kale, papaya, red bell pepper, brussels sprouts, asparagus, and lettuce.

Vitamin D is for normal growth and development of bones and teeth, as well as improved resistance against certain diseases. You can get natural vitamin D just by going outside and standing in the sun. That's right the sun heals your bones, teeth and protects you from viruses and diseases.

Folate/folic acid protects your body produce and maintain new cells, and it stops changes to DNA that may lead to cancer. As a healer, doctors prescribe it to treat folic acid deficiency and certain types of anemia (lack of red blood cells) due to lack of folic acid. Folic acid foods are leafy green vegetables, such as spinach, citrus fruits, beans, bread, rice, cereal, pasta, and wheat grain.

Iron is a mineral that is a necessity to the proper function of the hemoglobin. Hemoglobin is a protein needed to transport oxygen in the blood. Iron also has a role in a number of other important processes in the body. Lack of iron in the blood can lead to a range of serious health problems, including iron deficiency anemia

Selenium is important part to healing your immune system. This is an antioxidant that helps lower oxidative stress in your body, it reduces inflammation and enhances immunity. It has been proven throughout decades, maybe even a millennium. Selenium increase blood levels and are associated with enhanced immune response. Selenium foods are nuts, oats, beans lentil and Spanish.

Copper is a necessity for the anatomy. You can find copper in green leafy foods, dark chocolate, and beans.

Zinc is used for the proper growth and maintenance of the human body. Usually It is found in several systems and biological processes, and it is needed for immune function, wound healing, blood clotting, thyroid function, and much more. Zinc is said to also have effects against viruses. Foods with Zinc are nuts, lentil, beans and chickpeas

Vitamin B12 is good for the brain and DNA functions. Vitamin B12 foods are bananas, potatoes and spinach.

Vitamin K. It produces blood clotting, bone metabolism, and regulating blood calcium levels. Your body needs vitamin K in order to produce prothrombin. Prothrombin is a protein and clotting factor that is important in blood clotting and bone metabolism. Also Vitamin K is great for eye sight. This is what I consider an ultimate vital to the body. Vitamin K foods are kiwi, broccoli, asparagus, kale, cabbage family, spinach, turnip greens, blueberries, Leaf vegetables, okra, beans and sauerkraut.

Vitamin B6 benefits the central nervous system. It is involved in producing the neurotransmitters serotonin and norepinephrine, and in forming myelin. Also known as pyridoxine. This I essential vitamin is a water-soluble vitamin, which means it dissolves in water. Vitamin B6 foods are whole grain, vegetables and beans

Vitamin D comes naturally from the sun. It's a necessary component to Healing the body. Also potatoes contain vitamin D. Which also means sweet potatoes red potatoes and all other potatoes do too. Vitamin D heals your bones. Stay away from dairy meaning from animal do not drink from an animal it's meant for the animal there immune system is different from the human body and woman's body.

Niacin better commonly known as vitamin B3, is a necessity nutrient. In fact, every part of our body needs it to work properly. Niacin helps lower cholesterol, ease arthritis and boost brain function. Vitamin B3 foods are peanuts, sunflower seeds, avocado, potatoes, green peas, whole grain, brown rice, broccoli and unbleached flour.

Riboflavin (vitamin B2) helps break down proteins, fats, and carbohydrates. Vitamin B2 maintains the body's energy supply. In addition it helps convert carbohydrates into adenosine triphosphate. Adenosine triphosphate also abbreviated as ATP, is an energy-carrying molecule that is found in the cells of all living things. ATP captures chemical energy obtained from the breakdown of food molecules and releases it to fuel other cellular. B2 foods are almonds, avocado, spinach, asparagus, Leaf vegetables, kidney beans and bread.

Thiamine (vitamin B1) allows the body to use carbohydrates as energy. Vitamin B1 is essential for glucose metabolism. It's important in the functioning in the nerve, muscle, and heart vitals. Vitamin B12 foods are sunflower seeds, green peas, whole grains, bread, asparagus, brown rice, Lentil, potatoes, and kale.

Pantothenic acid (Vitamin B5) is one of the most vital vitamins for human life. It is important for making blood cells, and it helps you convert the food you eat into energy. Vitamin B5 is one of eight B vitamins. All B vitamins help you convert the protein, carbohydrates, and fats you eat into energy. Vitamin B5 foods are broccoli, avocado, shitake mushrooms, potatoes, lintel, peas, and raspberries.

Biotin is a vitamin that helps your body convert food into energy. It is also important during pregnancy and breastfeeding. This particular vitamin is important for the health of your hair, skin and nails. Foods that have biotin are sweet potatoes, almonds, avocado, spinach, nuts, and broccoli.

Invest in some Spirulina, its high protein green vegetables. This veggie high amounts of vitamins and nutrients. Spirulina offers antioxidant and inflammation-fighting highlights. It's said it's used to regulate the immune system.

THE AMAZING USES OF HONEY

Honey is one of the most powerful healing food sources ever created. Bees create honey through picking pollen from the beautiful flowers. Lucky for us the bees actually do what they were called to do. Honey heals the body in so many ways. It's used for allergies of all sorts. One example of allergies honey heals are pollen. Honey restores your immune system. It rebuilds your Anatomy. Honey cures common colds, viruses and diseases. Most important local honey (honey grown from the state and surrounding areas) makes your body a chameleon to the air.

According to research, eating honey may lead to modest reductions in blood pressure. It's an important risk factor for heart disease. Also honey is well known for its anti-inflammatory and antioxidant capacities, which may be useful for the prevention of chronic inflammatory process like atherosclerosis, diabetes mellitus and cardiovascular diseases. The antibacterial, anti-inflammatory and antioxidant properties of honey will be reviewed here on this particular site www.researchgate.net'

According to Healthline, honey promotes burn and wound healing. It has also been my personal experience honey healing my burn wound, it works.

Using the topical honey treatment has been used to heal wounds and burns since ancient times for an example early Kemet. Researchers have hypotheses saying that the honey healing powers comes from its antibacterial and anti-inflammatory effects as well as its ability to nourish surrounding tissue. Honey restores the vitals. It also used as a sweetener for teas, cakes brownies and other creative uses. Honey is a great superfood. Honey is an essential food to have in your home.

11 OILS CREATED FROM FRUITS AND VEGETABLES

E ucalyptus oil is available as an essential oil that is used as a medicine to treat a variety of common diseases and conditions including nasal congestion, asthma, and as a tick repellant. Diluted eucalyptus oil may also be applied to the skin as a remedy for health problems such as arthritis and skin ulcers.

Avocado Oil is rich in oleic acid is a very healthy fat. It reduces cholesterol and it improves heart health. Avocado Oil is high in lutein, an antioxidant that has benefits for the eyes. It also enhances the absorption of important nutrients and reduces symptoms of

Arthritis. Avocado Oil may even help prevent gum disease.

Benefits of Argan oil for skin ranges to many healing areas. Protects skin from burns. It moisturizes skin from becoming dry. Argan oil treats a number of skin conditions like acne, skin infections, and wounds. It also soothes atopic dermatitis. It has anti-aging effects. You can use it as a depository for hair growth. It's also edible and a good source of health benefits such as prevent chronic illnesses, including heart disease, diabetes, and cancer. It is an anti-inflammatory and a necessity to nutrients for the body.

Palm oil is used for preventing vitamin A deficiency, cancer, and brain disease. It's also used to heal aging skin. It treats malaria, high blood pressure, high cholesterol, and cyanide poisoning. Palm oil has been used for weight loss and increasing the body's metabolism. As food, palm oil is used for frying and other creative innovative cook accessory.

Olive oil is huge in healthy monounsaturated fats. It also contains large amounts of antioxidants. Olive

Oil has strong anti-Inflammatory characteristics that helps prevent strokes. Olive Oil is protective against heart disease. Olive oil is used for cooking and it's also used as dressings for salads and other cooking uses. It's also used to moisturize the scalp and also as a depository for hair growth.

Rosemary oil is used in aromatherapy. Rosemary Oil is amazing in reducing of stress levels and nervous tension. It builds mental activity. Rosemary encourages an insight, relieve fatigue, and support respiratory function. We use this herb to improve alertness, eliminate negative moods, and increase the retention of information by enhancing concentration. Rosemary is one of many Mediterranean herbs that have been used to cure a variety of illness such as, baldness or the gout. It's also is used to make breads and other creative chef ideas. It is also used to open the follicle in pores of the skin.

Thyme oil is created from the perennial herb known as Thymus vulgaris. The herb is a known as a mint. It's been used for cooking, mouthwashes, potpourri and aromatherapy. This oil has antiseptic, antibacterial, antispasmodic, hypertensive and has calming properties.

Thyme oil is anti-inflammatory. It's commonly used to preserve foods, cosmetics, and toiletries. It's also been found as an ingredient in mouthwash.

Marigold oil also known as the Calendula flower is used to prevent muscle spasms and the start menstrual periods. It reduces fever. It is also used for treating sore throat and mouth. It's used to ease pain of menstrual cramps, heals cancer, and stomach and duodenal ulcers. Calendula has also been used for measles, smallpox, and jaundice. Calendula oil has antifungal, anti-inflammatory, and antibacterial properties that might make it useful in healing wounds, soothing eczema, and relieving diaper rash. It's also used as an antiseptic. Marigold is mostly used and making soups, stews or you might even want to try as a salad.

Lemon oil is good for stimulating, calming, astringent, detoxifying, antiseptic, disinfectant, and getting rid of fungus.

Mandarin oil Promotes cellular growth. It has a high amount of vitamins, nutrients and antioxidants. Mandarin Essential Oil helps with producing new skin cells and tissues. This oil is used for detoxing. It has an anti-inflammatory property. It gives complete relief for the body and also improves blood circulation.

Peppermint oil good for lungs, it eliminate harmful bacteria, and relieves muscle spasms. Peppermint oil flatulence, disinfect and soothes skin that is inflamed.

Geranium oil reduce feelings of stress, anxiety, sadness, fatigue, and tension. It's also used for relaxation. It's also used to heal the skin and healthy hair. This oil calm nerves and reduce the feelings of stress. Geranium is also known to get rid of bothersome insects.

Rosemary good for lungs, It also encourages clarity and insight to concentrate. Rosemary opens up pores and relieve fatigue. Some uses it to help respiratory system function. It is used to improve alertness and eliminate negative moods. Rosemary oil increases the retention of information by enhancing focus.

Sage oil is used to heal bacterial infections, spasms, eliminate toxins. It also provides relief for digestive complaints, and calm skin conditions such as dermatitis and athlete's foot. This oil have antibacterial properties. Sage has a natural antidepressant. It relieves the pains of menopause symptoms and cramps.

Eucalyptus oil good for lungs and is an anti-inflammatory. The eucalyptus oil is antispasmodic, decongestant, and a healer for several functions of the body respiratory system. It can be used as a deodorant, and offers antiseptic qualities.

Lavender oil it's used to relax and calm nervous system. It's also has antiseptic and anti-inflammatory agents that help heal minor burns and bug bites. Lavender oil is also used for treating anxiety, insomnia, depression, and restlessness.

Basil oil is used as a muscular aches, spasms, gout, flatulence, and exhaustion. It is also known to enhance the immune system functions. It's also used to protect against infection, reduce water retention, and stabilize irregular menstruation patterns.

Chamomile oil heals the digestive system such as indigestion, nausea, or gas. Chamomile oil also heals wounds including ulcers and sores. It offers anxiety relief and easing skin conditions like eczema or rashes. Chamomile oil acts as an anti–inflammation and pain reliever for conditions like back pain, neuralgia, or arthritis. The most common use of chamomile oil is to promote sleep rest.

Vetiver is used for balancing, calming, and grounding self. It's commonly used to promote restful sleep and address restlessness. This oil is an anti-septic, anti-spasmodic, and immune-stimulating for the anatomy. It's also used as a sedative. It's stimulate circulation if blood. This oil has many ways of healing like, soothe feelings of anger, anxiety, exhaustion, irritability, and stress

Fennel oil is great as an antispasmodic, particularly for the digestive, cardiovascular and respiratory systems. It heals wounds. Boosts mental health and helps digestion system.

Sandalwood oil helps with disorders, including anxiety, bronchitis, diarrhea, fatigue, fever, and. gallbladder problems. It also heals high blood pressure, indigestion, insomnia, liver problems and low intimacy Drive. It's been known to heal sore throats and urinary tract issues.

Jojoba is also known as the Simmondsia Chinensis. Oil is also used as its seed. Jojoba beans are edible. The seed can be eaten raw or cooked but mostly boiled. The wax from the seed is used for skin in orders to alleviate the effects of psoriasis, sores, wounds and other skin afflictions. It has been used traditionally as a medicine for cancer, kidney disorders, colds, dysuria, obesity, parturition, aching eyes and warts, and to treat baldness.

Ylang Oil is an effective antidepressant, antiseptic and sedative. It heals the immune system health. It also contributes to proper blood flow and balance emotions. It makes a natural remedy for the endocrine plus the cardiovascular systems. A good susta of mine put me on to this oil. It helps with anatomy such as the reproductive and digestive systems.

Tonka Bean Oil can be used to make homemade remedies. We have been distracted but this natural oil helps increase sexual desire (as an aphrodisiac); and to treat menstrual cramps. Illnesses like stomach flu, cough, spasms, and tuberculosis don't stand a chance with Tonka bean oil.

Lavender Oil can be used to eliminate built up bacteria, muscle spasms, and relieve flatulence. This particular oil disinfects and heals irritated skin, bug bites and heals scars fast.

Gooseberries have a lot of fiber and is low in calories. It's good for its antioxidants. It's also been known to help control blood sugar. Gooseberries Works as a protector for the brain. It's been said to have some anti-cancer effects and is great boosters to heal the heart.

Aloe Vera Oil have many helpful healthy things to offer the anatomy. It offers Antioxidants and antibacterial healing. Heals burns vastly. Reduces dental plaque in mouth off teeth. Helps treat canker sores and improve skin. Helps with constipation and it prevent wrinkles.

Arnica Montana Oil helps to reduce inflammatory pain. Normally its used for the pain and swelling. Heals scars, muscle spasms, and stiff joint pain. It helps to boost circulation and speed up the skin healing. It also is safe and effective at easing pain.

Nettle oil works to relieve dry and a tense scalp. It's amazing for healing and growing hair especially for baldness in men and women. It's used to help flush toxins from the kidneys, and bladder function systems. Nettle tea is excellent for people who face bladder issues. It also helps balance excess sodium in the body makes a great detox.

Lavender oil heals by calming the nerves causing pain to be mild and allows body to relax

12 WHAT DO YOU KNOW ABOUT SALTS

Salts can be good and bad for the body. It could cause high blood pressure, high cholesterol or even heart attacks. What's not said is that all iodine salts are manipulated and bring no nutrition to the body unless you're trying to hurt yourself it weakens your immune system. I don't know if you've ever gave blood or plasma but they use iodine to thin out your skin to make your veins visible. Just imagine what it does for your insides. Hmm, makes you think right. Well salts that are amazing and helps replenish your body entirely are sea salts.

Sea salts from different areas varies but they are good for the body's nutrition and immune system. Sea salt is mostly composed of sodium chloride.

Sodium chloride is a compound that helps regulate fluid balance and blood pressure in the body. Sea salt contains some minerals, including potassium, iron, and calcium. Vital minerals like sodium, chloride, potassium, calcium, magnesium, copper, zinc among other beneficial trace elements. This is in comparison to table salt who only have only sodium chloride.

A great sea salt to use is Himalayan salt. It is rock salt mined from the Punjab region of Pakistan. This salt normally has a pink salt. It is commonly used as a food additive as table salt. It can be used as a material for cooking, food flavoring, and spa treatments. Himalayan salt contains more calcium, potassium, magnesium and iron than many salts. This just a personal favorite of mine and many others but is a wide range of brands and geographic to choose from.

Different foods that produce collagen for the body varies. Broccoli, brussels sprouts, red peppers, oranges, and kale are all examples of just some of the citrus fruits vegetables and leafy greens that put back into the collagen of the body. Vegetables such as leafy greens beans and avocado put in a high amount of Replacements to add back to your collagen. Also you can get the same results with berries, garlic and citrus fruits. In taking vegetables and fruits, considering it all heals the body way quicker and way more accurately than anything else is amazing. The beauty of it is that you can literally go buy seeds and plant them right in your own backyard. It's something like a fountain of youth right fruits and vegetables.

It's time for our people to realize that you can absolutely heal yourself with different foods, vegetables and herbs.

Due to the fact that a lot of us are not scientists, we don't really trip off of our blood types. It's very much important in order to know what it is your missing in your body and what type of diet you must customize your body to. Throughout the millennium's, blood types have separated into several different categories. It's an absolute, to alert yourself of what your body needs and of your families. It has become most imperative that we start analyzing and building our anatomy with putting the right vitas into your body. These particular vitals are found in a variety of vegetables, fruits and herbs. Your body consistently heals naturally. All that that you intake into your body determines if it's going to work correctly as it should. Build your anatomy, it's amazing to be able to.

WORDS FROM AUTHOR

Please note never forget that the trees grant us oxygen air grants us nitrogen and all of the elements around us these are all Necessities to life. You may have foods that grow right outside your door that you do not even sure of. We all have a part in The Grand Design, research, it couldn't do anything but help.

It's important to know your blood type and the vitals that need to be strengthened. You can replace what is missing from your anatomy with different fruits, veggies herbs and spices. All can survive it's just a matter of doing your personal research on self for self or even others. Build positive bonds with people like minds and others all need each other.

We can rebuild all that has been lost within us. It's time to heal. Each one teach one.

It's most interesting how much of our families eat these items anyway and never think of how strong they are for our bodies in our immune system. We heal ourselves from illnesses not even knowing so. Using this fun fact packet you should now embark on healing your families from viruses, illnesses and diseases that bring nothing but death amongst our people we will get through this together. Together we will rise as healthy energetic creative an illness free peoples.

-Jerrica Whittier